Matters of the Heart

Thank you for your support

Love Denise

Matters of the Heart

My Journey Surviving 10 years and 5 months on the Heart Transplant List

Dennis Thomas

As told to

Nicol McClendon

Matters of the Heart

My Journey Surviving 10 years and 5 months on the Heart Transplant List

Published by NM Publishing – Candy's Legacy
www.nicolmcclendon.com

Manuscript Editing
Pamela Mobley - Thompson

ISBN for Paperback: 978-1-7359046-0-3

Printed in the United States of America

In Loving Memory of

my grandmother

Willa Mae "Aunt Babe" Moreland Womack

June 30, 1926 – December 8, 2009

"A medical condition is not a tragedy. It is a mindset that is overcome by education, support and the will to get better."

Dennis Thomas February 1, 2019

B efore I ever touched a basketball, baseball was my sport of choice. However, the summer between my last year of junior high school and my freshman year of high school, I had a growth spurt of four or five inches. Standing six-foot-one, I tried out and made the school's freshman basketball team.

I wasn't new to playing basketball. When I was young, my grandfather built and installed a basketball hoop in the driveway of our family home. He used a fence post and shaped the backboard out of wood. He also found a used net for a hoop. Once he was done, we had a mini basketball court. The driveway court became a place for my neighborhood friends and me to hang out and shoot hoops. We would spend hours every day playing ball. We had to play one on one as the driveway was not big enough for more than two of us to play at a time. So, one on one was the game we played until everyone had a chance to play. The first player to reach five points was the winner. The winner stayed in the game until they lost.

In high school, we frequented Bloomfield's Rockwell Park. That was our area's version of New York City's, The Rucker Park, the most famous outdoor basketball court in America. Rockwell was where my friends and I would play games of five on five. Rockwell was also the destination for the best basketball players in our area to play, both old and young. At that time, our five included me and my best friends, Phil and Tone, our friend Lorenzo and Phil's stepfather, "Big O." We would walk up to the court and ask, "Who got next?" Once it was our turn, we stayed on the court for hours because we were always winning. We would also travel around the state to play at different courts. "Big O," being the oldest, was the designated driver. Since we were playing the best of the best at these parks, this experience allowed us to keep getting better at the game we loved.

Street ball was different from organized ball. We learned how to be tough and fearless. Everyone knew we were fierce opponents who played with heart. We also learned that you must depend on your team, and everyone had to contribute something in order to win.

Basketball helped develop my social skills. Being a good ball player built your reputation. Simply put, when people respected your game, they usually respected you. Basketball was also an excellent networking vessel; I have built some lifelong friendships and connections playing the game I love. I had no idea how desperately I would need many of those relationships later in life.

After high school I went to trade school to be an electrician. I finished the electrical program and obtained my certificate. While looking for work as an electrician, a family friend recommended me for a job as a construction laborer. Here I was, a single, young Black man, making good money. Being a laborer afforded me my first real opportunity at independence when I was able to purchase my first car. I felt like I was on top of the world. But, as luck would have it, I was laid off a year later due to a work shortage.

Newly unemployed, another friend advised me of a local daycare looking for male teachers. I applied and was hired as a part time teacher's aide. Within three months I was promoted to full time. I was told for me to advance I would need to obtain my certification. I applied and was accepted into Capital Community College, where they were offering a free Early Childhood Education certification program. I made the Dean's list every semester and completed the program. Upon completion, I obtained state certification and was promoted to head teacher, with my very own classroom. Talk about ecstatic and proud!

For a 19-year-old Black male, this was a huge accomplishment. I loved nurturing, mentoring and building relationships with the children and their families. I taught the kids to respect each other and never give up.

My classroom motto was "Always be a step ahead of others." Many of the children in my classroom did not have strong male role models in their lives. So aside from their daily learning, I taught many of them basic life skills, like how to tie their shoes. I stressed the importance of teamwork. I also taught them to have routines and the benefits of healthy eating. And of course, we played sports. When we were able to go outside, teaching them basketball skills and dodge ball was my favorite activity. I loved my job and I loved those kids, so much so, I taught preschool for twelve years.

In my free time, I coached boys ages 14-17 in the Amateur Athletic Union (AAU) Basketball Program. We practiced all year and traveled to different gyms in the Tri-state area (Connecticut, Massachusetts and New York) to play in tournaments. Of course, I loved basketball and coaching provided me the opportunity to help young boys increase their knowledge and love of the game as well as, hone in on their skills on and off the court. AAU provided exposure for the kids to play against different teams similar to what I had at Rockwell Park. It also gave the kids who wanted to play on a collegiate level or professionally, the opportunity to perfect their skills. We also worked with the kids on the skills they lacked or areas of weakness to help them make their high school teams and become student athletes, with *student* being the operative word. We always reinforced the importance of education.

By this time, I was 30 years old with a good career and a hobby that I loved. I worked at the preschool and coached until August 9, 2009.

4

August 8, 2009

I have a close-knit family, so naturally, we watch out for each other. Any given Sunday you would find us fellowshipping at someone's house, enjoying each other's company, and eating a good meal. Usually we could tell when something wasn't quite right with one of us. On this particular Sunday, we were at my sister's house. My body was feeling a little run down, however I simply felt it was the residual effects of a cold from the week before. As we sat in the kitchen, my mom looked at me and mentioned that I did not look well. I told her that the week prior I had what I thought was a common cold. The symptoms were slowly progressing to flu like symptoms and I was experiencing fatigue from lack of sleep. I also had a cough that I couldn't get rid of. She recommended that I go to the hospital for a checkup.

August 9, 2009

As usual, I went to work at the preschool. I called my doctor's office to set up an appointment and he scheduled it for that day at lunch time. When I arrived, my primary care doctor was not there. I saw a covering doctor who, upon examination, informed me that he believed I had a blood clot in my lungs and immediately sent me to the Emergency Room at Hartford Hospital. He called ahead to advise them I was coming and that I would need a CAT scan. I drove straight to the Emergency Room with my paperwork and waited to be seen. Within the next few hours, I had chest x-rays and was scheduled for a CAT scan. I called my job and advised them I would not be returning for the day. After the CAT scan, I called my mom and immediate family members, informed them of my status and kept them abreast of my treatment. Within an hour, my mom, brother and sister had arrived at the hospital. About 10:00 p.m., we were informed that I was being admitted for additional testing. The next day I continued to have more diagnostic testing. One of the tests even required me to be sedated under general anesthesia.

After waking up, I found myself hooked up to IV's and oxygen pumps. To my surprise, I was in the Intensive Care Unit. I was told a doctor would be in to speak with me. The doctor arrived and informed me that I was in heart failure and they were awaiting results from my diagnostic tests to decide if I was a candidate for a heart transplant or a heart mate.

My doctor stated, "A heart transplant is a surgical transplantation procedure that is performed on patients suffering from severe coronary artery disease or end-stage heart failure. A functioning heart from a recently deceased organ donor is implanted into a patient when other medical or surgical treatments have failed to suffice. It is not considered a cure, but a life-saving treatment that is intended to improve the chances of survival and provide a better quality of life to individuals. Patients who do not qualify for a heart transplant may be prescribed a left ventricular assist device (LVAD) or an artificial heart. Nearly 3,500 heart transplant surgeries are performed worldwide every year. The survival period post-operation at the time is averaged to be at ten years."

That was a lot of information to digest. I was confused as to why my heart was failing. It didn't make sense. I was young and healthy. I was an athlete with no prior medical issues. As you can imagine, I was devastated by this news.

While hospitalized and waiting for my test results, I was started on a regimen of medication. Lots of medication. The plan was to stabilize the remaining functioning of my heart. I started taking ten pills with IV medications around the clock. I also had to have a Swan catheter inserted in my neck.

The Swan is a measuring device inserted in the right side of the heart. Its job was to log and keep track of the pulmonary artery pressure. The Swan would need to be changed weekly.

Immediately after the Swan was implanted, I was so weak. I only had the physical capacity to walk from the bed to the chair in my hospital room. Now, not only did my body have to adjust to the medication that I was receiving, but I also had to adjust to being connected to an IV Pole 24 hours a day.

The first two weeks in the hospital were like being on a medically and physically exhausting roller coaster. I had some good days and then there were days when I was in a lot of physical pain. My mental state also took a beating.

Most of the physical pain I experienced was from the catheter attachment that was stitched to my neck for the Swan device. During the first week in the hospital, there were so many tests like, EKG's and blood work ups. Sometimes I felt like a rag doll. After the first week, there was an attempt to wean me off some of the medication. The plan was to slowly taper down the medications to the lowest dosage. However, once the medical team started to taper the meds, my blood pressure dropped so low that I became fatigued and had to go back up to the highest dosage.

Also, during this time, my heart failure team was assembled, and I was introduced to my surgeon. It was a Wednesday night when the surgeon visited me for the first time to discuss my options.

Application for a heart

I felt like I was being interviewed and the application for a heart was the interviewer.

Do you want a heart with a Leaky valve? A heart with Hepatitis A, B? HIV? Do you want to wait for the perfect heart? Can you wait? Will you survive the wait? How about a mechanical heart with the hope of going home while waiting for a heart? Are you a candidate for a Heartmate Left Ventricular Assist Device (LVAD/VAD)?

A Heartmate LVAD/VAD is a mechanical pump that helps hearts that aren't pumping adequately, to push the right amount of blood throughout the body. It is attached to your heart. The damaged part of your heart would be removed and replaced with the Heartmate.

After the application for the heart and my discussion with the surgeon, he said I had 24 hours to think about my contract to a new lease on life. He also indicated that the heart team and committee meet on Thursdays to discuss options for current patients.

24 hours to make a decision. Whoa!

This is the time when I needed my support system. I needed to have a real heart to heart with those closest to me, the ones who had always been in my corner, through the good and the bad.

Before the surgeon left, he recommended I watch a video that would provide insight and help me gain some clarity as I weighed my options. It would be a long night.

After considering all your options, you make a decision. However, it is the heart team and committee that reviews all of your medical information and ultimately makes the final decision.

My surgeon returned the next night. It was a Thursday. He advised me that as my test results were being reviewed, it became clear that I was not a candidate for a Heartmate. My heart was too damaged and I would need a new heart. I was also too high risk to be discharged while awaiting a new heart.

My decision was made for me.

After all the contemplating, playing out the different scenarios in my head, and the exhausting mental showdown between my head and my heart (no pun intended), eventually, someone, other than me, got the final say. And then, you wait!

Ironically, praying for a miracle means hoping someone dies so you can live.

The mental anguish I experienced while trying to navigate through a plethora of thoughts and emotions was overwhelming and exhausting. Add that with having to come to terms with my quickly declining health and strength, and it's a wonder I didn't lose my mind right then and there.

Every week when The Swan was replaced, my anxiety went into overdrive. This was the mental part of the roller coaster. It was a mental battle I thought would get better, but as time went on, the anxiety became progressively worse. It was so bad that I needed a sedative on the days of my procedure. Unfortunately, the mental suffering wasn't the only side effect. On the day of the procedure and the following 24 hours, you're not allowed to walk. Your body had to readjust every time the catheter was replaced, and resting was necessary for an accurate reading of your pulmonary function. This started over every week. Baseline. My body would be weak for days after the procedure. But, no sooner than my strength came back, the process started all over again.

After the first two weeks on the medically and physically exhausting roller coaster, my surgeon returned. He told me it was my responsibility to follow all of the directions given by the medical team and to keep up my strength. Simply put, I had to stay healthy.

At the time, I couldn't understand how it was *my* responsibility to stay healthy since I was in a hospital, surrounded by people who had taken an oath to save lives. I thought it was *their* responsibility to keep me healthy. I soon found out that my responsibilities were to move, to not get sick and to stay put in the hospital.

He went on to tell me that it was his responsibility to find me the best heart. I told him I would hold him to that.

According to the medical team's directions, staying in bed all day was a no-no! With the medical staff's assistance, I was expected to walk around the ICU floor several times a day.

11

This restriction was due to my fatigue with The Swan device and the weekly procedures to change it.

I immediately started setting small goals for myself. My first goal was to build-up my physical strength enough to walk on my own and be allowed to walk to and around the adjacent units. I walked daily and it wasn't long before I reached my goal. Four weeks had gone by and my medical team was proud of my progress and trusted the fact that I was committed to staying healthy. They believed in me just as much as I believed in myself.

After the first four weeks, I was getting stronger every day. Every morning the medical team would do their rounds and they had determined I was stabilizing. No, not enough to leave the hospital, but enough to survive the wait for a heart, if I kept up my walking routine. They also advised me that if I remained stable, I could sit outside and get some fresh air. How many times had I taken fresh air for granted? The one and only time I was able to sit outside during my hospital stay was in October 2009. This was a wonderful gift. 20 minutes outside. It felt so good to be outside however, it would be the last time until I was discharged from the hospital.

Home life before admission

Before being admitted to the hospital, I was so full of life. I was also a loving grandson who cherished the close relationship my grandmother and I shared. Our bond was solid and special. We lived together for a few years before my grandmother had an accident in the house. She fell one day and was hospitalized. She was then transferred to a rehabilitation facility. I would visit her every day prior to my own hospitalization. I would work from 7:00 a.m. to 3:00 p.m. then visit her. I would bring her favorite snacks, Almond Joys and orange soda. We would talk about life and how I was doing. She would always ask me if I was taking care of the house. We talked about basketball. While my grandmother didn't watch a lot of the games, she absolutely loved the drafts. She would say, "It was so wonderful to see those boys, most straight out of high school fulfilling their dreams and having the opportunity at a better life." We would sit and watch some of her favorite TV shows which included the news.

After I was admitted, she called me every day. She said she just wanted to make sure I was OK. We even received special permission for her to visit me. She was able to visit three times during my hospitalization; September 13, 2009, once in October 2009 and our final visit was in early November 2009.

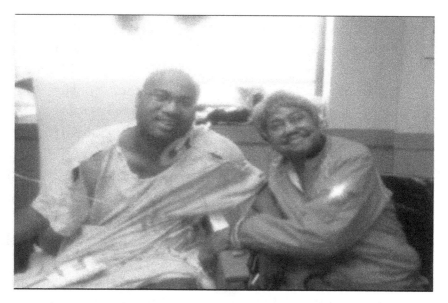

I didn't know that the visit in early November would be my last time seeing her. She was supposed to visit me on my birthday, however, they said she was unable to come. At the time, no one told me the reason she couldn't visit me, but I later learned that my grandmother's health had started to decline.

Still waiting on a heart

My birthday, November 23, 2009, was the last time I spoke to my grandmother. Although she wasn't able to come and see me, she did call to wish me a happy birthday. She said she wasn't feeling well. It would be the last time I heard her voice.

By now, I had been in the hospital for three months. My family threw me a surprise birthday party in the hospital's family room. About thirty of my family and friends, and some medical staff were there. They shut down the family visiting suite to accommodate my party. I was beyond happy. It was the first time in a long time that I was able to feel some sense of normalcy. However, the hospital gown and IV pole were constant reminders that normal was a bit of a stretch. It didn't matter though because I was surrounded by love.

Unfortunately, my grandmother's health continued to decline. She passed away two weeks later on December 8, 2009.

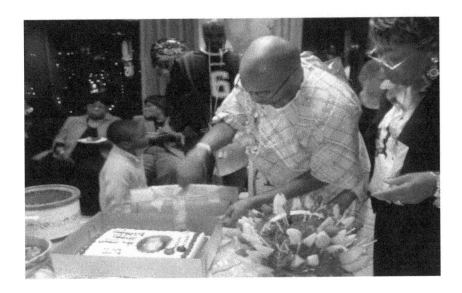

Life in the hospital

Being hospitalized for a long period of time takes some getting used to. My routine included waking up at 7:00 a.m. for the switch of the nursing staff. Luckily, I had the same nursing team, so we became used to each other. I was familiar with my team and they became my family. However, even though they were becoming like family, I still was not comfortable with my new life in the hospital. In addition to the Swan's continuous connection to my neck, the IV pole with countless fluid changes, the cuff checking my blood pressure every hour on the hour, the nightly blood draws and/or every time the doctor requested, the having to buzz for assistance to get out of bed and use the bathroom every time I needed to relieve myself (I had restrictions so bathroom checks were mandatory), the constant bells and whistles from the monitors (both mine and the other patients in the ICU), I was extremely restless. Even though the lights in my room were dim, my sleep pattern was off. I couldn't sleep more than 30 minutes at any given time.

To pass the time and find some semblance of comfort, my hospital room became a small apartment. The room came equipped with the standard small 12" hospital TV; however, the nursing staff requested a larger TV for me. They had a cart rolled in with a 27" TV and a DVD player. They even had the cable that was hooked up to the smaller TV connected to the larger TV so I could have access to all channels. My family also bought me a laptop and I had access to the Internet via the hospital's Wi-Fi. I had a table full of snacks, books, magazines and newspapers. I also had a trophy on the table.

That year the team I had been coaching before my hospital stay, won the championship game. The coach said the team was down 15 points at half time. During his halftime speech, he asked them, "What would Coach Dennis do?" The team was motivated and rallied back in the second half to win the chip. They insisted that I have the trophy.

I had many visitors. Most days I would have visits two to three times a day. In addition to my family supporting and visiting me, some of my most memorable visits were from my longtime friend Bob. He visited me every Sunday and always brought the Sunday newspaper. We would talk and reminisce about the old times and how things would be once I received my new heart and was able to leave the hospital. This encouraged me and kept me hopeful looking toward the future.

My Barber also visited me and provided a free haircut every Friday morning.

Other transplant recipients

I had my own room and was also now free to walk about the ICU while most of the other ICU patients were bed bound. Some were also waiting for organs to receive transplants. Not just for new hearts but for just about every organ imaginable. I would often go to the other rooms to interact with them. During my walks I would also meet many of their families.

There was another heart failure patient in ICU waiting for a transplant. We would talk often during our hospital stay. During one of our many conversations, I mentioned to him that I had never been fishing but always wanted to go. He promised me that after we received our new hearts, recovered, were released from the hospital and healthy enough to go, he would bring me fishing. As luck would have it, he received his heart two days before mine. He kept his promise and six months after my release, he took me fishing with his daughter. We had bonded on a level that only heart transplant recipients could even understand. We knew the journey and patience it took to wait for a new heart. We bonded during our fishing trip and I thought we would be friends for the remainder of our lives. Sadly, a year after our fishing trip, his daughter called me with the worst news. My friend, fishing buddy and transplant brother had passed away.

During my hospital stay, I became close with an older gentleman who was also waiting on a heart. I was walking around the ICU one day and walked past his room. He yelled out, "You're burning a hole in the floor!" I assumed he was referring to my nonstop walking. At the time he was able to walk, but I later learned he was no longer motivated to do so. During my walks, stopping by his room became part of my daily routine. I would encourage him to take small steps and ask for help when needed. He started walking again and we became walking buddies. Every morning we would walk together. He would say walking together made him feel better. He later introduced me to his son and daughter. They expressed their appreciation for me looking after their dad and keeping his spirits up while they were not around. One morning I went to his room for our usual walk. When I walked into his room, he said he wasn't feeling well and that we would walk together later on in the day. I did a short walk and returned to my room to rest up for our longer walk when he was able to join me. Later that day I told my nurse I was ready for my afternoon walk but she told me I couldn't leave my room at that time. She said no patients were allowed in the hallway or out of their rooms. A few minutes later my walking buddy's son and daughter came in my room. I could tell they had been crying. They thanked me for everything I had done for their father, especially for being his friend, a listening ear and motivating him to push through his pain. After them expressing their gratitude for my friendship with their dad, they finished by saying "Sadly our dad passed away a few moments ago." They left my room and I sat there speechless. That moment changed my life.

His passing could have easily defeated someone in my situation; a situation not identical, but very similar to his. I was waiting on a heart and doing everything I could to stay healthy while waiting. However, instead of feeling defeated or fearful, I began to pray harder. I continued to walk and keep the faith. His children's gratitude fueled me. I wanted to continue helping others. It made me work harder to build my strength and as I continued to walk, I introduced myself to others along the journey. I started encouraging and motivating everyone I encountered. I would tell them to stay strong and keep hope alive.

Soon the word began to spread about my mentoring and visits with other patients. My constant walking also had me strong enough that I no longer needed assistance during my walks.

My story ended up reaching the CEO of Hartford Hospital. One day I was out walking and as I was heading back to my room, I noticed a gentleman standing in front of my door. It turns out, he was looking for me and waiting on my return. He introduced himself and said he had heard a lot about me. He wanted to meet me and get to know more about me. As we sat and talked, we discovered that we shared a love for basketball. He also let me know he was proud of me as a patient and appreciated the mental fortitude it took for me to encourage others while I was also waiting for a heart. Before he departed, he said he would keep in touch. He would call often and check up on me to see how I was holding up. Unfortunately, I didn't see him again until the day I was released from the hospital.

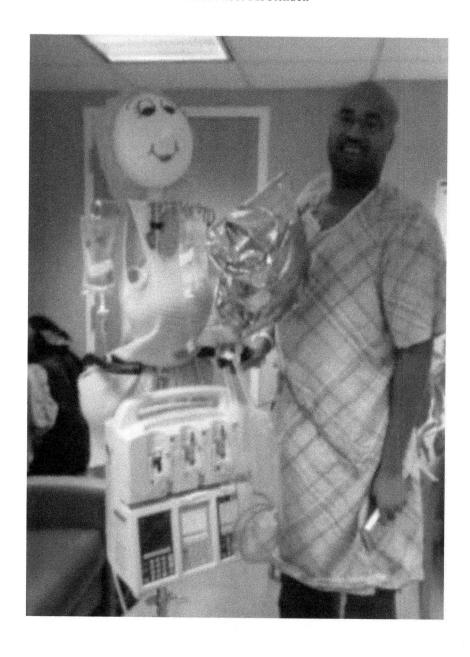

Grieving

Knowing how close my grandmother and I were, my family had to decide on whether or not to tell me about her declining health and passing. They knew how fragile I was, emotionally and physically. They also knew how the whole situation was starting to take its toll on me. So, in a collaborative effort by my family and medical team to spare me any additional trauma and stress, my family decided not to tell me about my grandmother. I found out almost a week later. Knowing that I was unable to see her one last time before her passing was a torturous nightmare.

My grandmother's funeral was scheduled for December 14, 2009.

My family and I requested special approval for me to leave the hospital and have a private viewing at the church. I needed to grieve and seeing her one last time would help. One of my nurses and a respiratory therapist volunteered to accompany me, however the hospital declined our request. My family decided they would record the service and we would have a viewing in the hospital chapel.

That would never happen.

December 12, 2009

At 5:30 in the morning, I was awakened by my nurse. She said, "They've found you a heart." I was half asleep but I sat up in disbelief and put on my glasses. As the room came into focus, I was able to see a wondrous sight. Every nurse on third shift was standing in front of my door crying. It was at that moment, I knew it was true. My new heart was on its way. My first thought was my surgeon had kept his promise. He had, indeed, found me the best heart.

I couldn't wait to call my family and tell them the good news.

My first call was to my Uncle Paul. He was like a father to me. He had moved into the family home that I once shared with my grandmother. I told him my new heart was on the way. He was overcome with emotion and shared with me that a few moments before my call, the old quartz clock in the living room started to spin and chime. This clock, which was encased in glass, had a gold angel that would spin every time the clock struck a new hour. It would chime so loudly. Ironically, the clock didn't have a battery in it and had not worked in years. He said as soon as the clock started spinning and chiming, the phone rang, and it was me with my good news.

We praised God! He and I both knew it was a sign from my grandmother. I'm sure she was smiling and watching over me as I vowed to make the most out of my second chance at life.

December 13, 2009

Finally! On the day of surgery, my family came to visit and celebrate my new beginning. Because my grandmother's homegoing service was scheduled for the day after my surgery, there were so many family members in town. I had visitors coming and going all day. Everyone was so happy that the day had finally come. Overjoyed was an understatement. Although everyone was grieving the loss of our matriarch, we celebrated my chance at a second lease on life.

My doctor was in route to Philadelphia to harvest my new heart. All day doctors were coming in and out checking on me. My medication was adjusted, and I was being weaned off all the medication I had been taking to stabilize my heart in preparation for surgery. I couldn't walk around because the Swan that had been attached to me for months, was now being prepped for removal. The last of my blood work was being checked to ensure compatibility with my soon to be arriving new heart.

My new heart finally arrived and at 8:30 pm, I was in surgery. By 11:15 pm, the surgery was complete, and I was placed on life support. On December 13, 2009 at 11:45 pm, I was breathing on my own and off life support.

Waking up after surgery, I was in a lot of pain but thankful to be among the living and excited about a promising future. First, it was a relief to wake up. You pray and hope for the best during surgery and when you open your eyes and realize you are still on top of the soil instead of under it, words can't completely grasp that feeling. After all the time spent in the hospital, waiting and then to finally be rewarded with a new heart, I immediately began thinking about the work needed in the upcoming days, weeks, months and years to remain strong and healthy. I knew there was a risk of rejection and I needed to make sure that the risk was slim to none. In life there are no guarantees and this life altering event was no different. So, the thought of complications was real. But I was already defying the odds by waking up, breathing on my own and completely off life support so soon after surgery. I wanted to speak so badly but the tubes down my throat made that an impossible feat. The nurse came in and saw that I was awake. My tubes were removed, and I gasped for air. My throat was raspy and dry. I needed fluid. My first precious words were used to ask for water.

December 14, 2009

My first visitors after surgery were my mom and my brother. They came to see me before my grandmother's funeral. I had written a letter just before my surgery to be read at the funeral. My brother agreed to read it and at the end, he was able to share the news of my successful surgery with the family. Even in our grief, there was a reason to rejoice.

Things moved pretty fast the first few days after surgery. Although the ICU on the 10th floor had been my home for the last four and a half months, I was moved to the ICU on the 9th floor of the hospital for the first few days after surgery. I was then moved out of ICU to the Step-Down Unit for continued observation, and after another few days, I was moved to my final home, the recovery room on the 9th floor. When I arrived at the recovery room, I was able to get up and walk around again.

I immediately asked every doctor and nurse that visited me, what I needed to do to leave the hospital. I also wanted to know how soon I would be released. My thoughts were consumed with leaving the hospital. I now had my new heart and I was ready to go home; I had been there long enough. However, before I could be released, I was told that I would be introduced to my new medication regimen. I had to learn all about the eighty new pills I was required to take daily. Yep, 8-0!!

This medication was my new normal and it was imperative that I become an expert on the very things that ultimately had the power to prolong my life or cut it short. All my medications, what time to take each pill, which ones I could mix and the ones I could not mix, were explained to me. I told my nurse I would know everything there was to know in three days. That was Friday, December 18, 2009.

Monday morning my nurse came in and gave me a test on my medication. Of course, I passed. I knew my medications inside and out. My nurse said he would consult with my doctors and I would be advised about a potential release day once it was determined.

December 21, 2009

During my walk around the unit, I saw my name on the board. My name was always there but this time there was an asterisk by it. That asterisk meant I was going home or at least I had a release date, December 24, 2009.

I was overcome with joy and the excitement felt like I had hit the lottery. Actually, I guess I had hit the lottery! Now don't get me wrong, receiving a new heart was definitely the jackpot but going home was the icing on the cake.

December 24, 2009

I paced the floor so much the night before that I could not sleep and now the day had come. I was giddy and scared. I was optimistic and cautious. I was elated and concerned. I was a bag of jumbled emotions. The last four and a half months consumed my entire being. I was excited about finally going home, however, I knew that I wasn't going back to the life I had before. I was also nervous and filled with fear of what my new life would be like. I wasn't returning to the house I once shared with my grandmother. I wasn't returning to the job I once loved. I wasn't returning to the basketball court to coach. I wasn't returning to the social life that I once had.

Your body has natural defenses it uses to protect itself from disease. After a life-saving heart transplant, your body tries to fight off what it thinks is a germ. It goes into attack mode to fight off this new potential threat. My new heart was at risk of being rejected by my body. So, to prevent a possible rejection I was required to take immunosuppressant medications. That meant I had to ward off not only a potential rejection, but also any infections. Being immunocompromised now meant that I would be quarantined for some time. Although I was going home, I'd still be confined to a certain extent, similar to the last four and a half months in the hospital. As much as I missed my home life, my responsibility now was to stay healthy and every move I made had a direct impact on the success or failure of my new heart.

The time had come. My mom, brother, sister and aunt arrived to bring me home. Once my room, my home for the last four and a half months, was all packed up and my release papers were signed, I was ready to go. I wanted to make sure I said my goodbyes to everyone I had met and everyone that had taken care of me during my hospital stay. However, I was told before I could leave someone special wanted to see me, so I had to wait. A few moments later, the CEO of the hospital arrived with a camera crew in tow.

Although we hadn't seen each other since his first visit, I remembered him as soon as I saw him walk into my room. He said because of the inspiration and motivation I had shown during my stay while waiting on my heart, he wanted to thank me for being so positive and a model patient. His present was documenting my departure. So, my family and I, along with the CEO and the camera crew, began my departure and descent from my room.

However, before we could head down to the lobby, we had to head up to my original home in the ICU on the 10th floor. I started my rounds saying my goodbyes to the patients, just as I had done on the 9th floor. Then we made our way to the door.

The next day was the best holiday ever.

December 25, 2009

That year my present was waking up at home. It wasn't about the gifts under the tree. More importantly, it was about the gift of life.

30

Life at home

The first seven years after my transplant were difficult. The transition from once being an independent free spirit, having no medical problems, with high energy and in my prime at 30 years old, to now a medication dependent person living with my family, was not easy.

I was overwhelmed at times. I was once young, athletic and fast. Now I weighed more than I ever had, and I was much slower than I had ever been. My new routine included cardiac rehabilitation three times a week to build my strength. My job was to learn my new body and my new heart. Always at the forefront of my mind was that I signed a contract for a new heart and the fine print was to obey the rules and stay healthy.

When I did regain my strength enough to work in some capacity, due to my immune system, I was unable to return to my day job working closely with small children. I also had not regained the level of energy required to run around a day care.

I was, however, still young enough for some resemblance of a normal life and I desired a love life.

After my transplant, I dated for a while and I did have one long term relationship where I was close to being in love. However, with my medical condition, I was unable to work a full-time job and earn a living close to what I once had. Working odd jobs was not enough to contribute to the household. Although I did give what I could and helped in many other ways, that was not enough. I earned just enough to have some level of independence and the hardest part was worrying about money. Lacking the ability to be the bread winner in the relationship hindered our future together. The expectation was that I stayed healthy, but I was stressing mentally and feeling the pressure.

Early 2017

I was at work one morning and felt sick. I ran to the bathroom and vomited. My job sent me home and I drove straight to the hospital. I knew something was wrong. I was admitted to the hospital directly through the Emergency Room. This time my stay was only three days. Once I was released, I was told I could not return to work. My cardiologist called a few days after, advising me I needed to come in for a visit.

On the day of the visit with my cardiologist, he explained I would need to be put back on the transplant list but first I needed to have a defibrillator implanted to keep track of my heart rate.

A defibrillator is a device that restores a normal heartbeat by sending an electric pulse or shock to the heart.

Defibrillators can also restore the heart's beating if the heart suddenly stops.

My new heart was at risk of stopping. Its functioning was slowly deteriorating.

July 5, 2017

I had the surgery to have the defibrillator implanted and by early 2018, after all my blood tests and medical work ups, I was placed back on a heart transplant list.

Something else happened in early 2018, I found the love of my life.

Although I was back on the transplant list, my life was starting to feel normal again, but for some reason I knew it would never be the same.

January 23, 2019

I had been having some weakness and fatigue. I advised my doctor of my symptoms and one of the tests he ordered was a colonoscopy. I assumed this was a precautionary measure. My new love and I went in the morning of the procedure. She said she would drop me off and await my call to pick me up. I was prepped for the procedure and put under general anesthesia. When I woke up, I wasn't expecting to see her but there she sat with tears in her eyes.

The only thing running through my mind was she was my second chance at love. I was so happy to have her. As I watched her closely, I realized that she was speaking to the doctor. Although I wasn't completely coherent, I clearly heard her when she looked at me and said, "Cancer."

Chemotherapy Day 1 - February 18, 2019

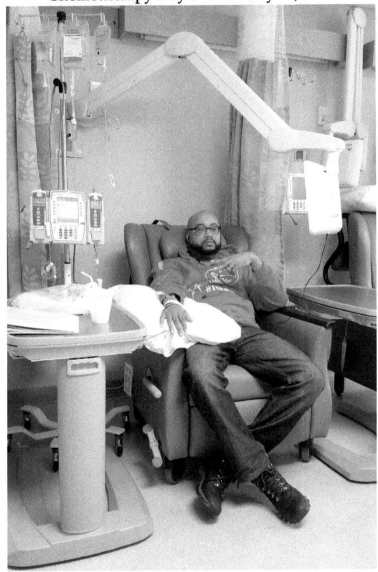

Dennis Thomas & Nicol McClendon

Matters of the Heart

Excerpt from *He Said/She Said: A Second Chance at Love*

By Nicol McClendon and Dennis Thomas

Coming 2021

He said:

"A new journey may begin with pain, but it ends with victory."

She said:

"After my darkest storm, I found something I thought I would never have again. Real love. The kind of love so strong that the smallest indiscretion sideswipes you and knocks you off your feet.

Today felt like that darkest storm, it rolled in quietly. The aftermath left me stunned. The hardest thing was trying to figure out how to put everything destroyed back to together and replace everything that was lost.

The thing about a sideswipe is you spend days thinking about what could have been done differently. How you could have prevented it from ever happening in the first place. You become obsessed with thinking about the things you can or can't do, to prevent it from ever happening again.

Life has a way of sideswiping you."

Dennis Thomas & Nicol McClendon

About the Authors

Dennis Thomas

Dennis Thomas is a sports enthusiast, basketball coach and former basketball player known for having a mean "pick". Dennis describes himself as a motivator.

He was a preschool teacher for twelve years and during this time, his love for mentoring and nurturing children continued to grow.

In 2009, Dennis became a heart transplant recipient. Today Dennis is celebrating ten years being a survivor.

He continues to mentor children in the community, on and off the court, via his work with Legacy Foundation of Hartford, Impact Training and Bulkeley High School.

Dennis visits Hartford Hospital often, counseling adults preparing for and recovering from organ transplants. He is also the "go-to" person many in the community call to counsel, support and encourage their loved ones through their own heart failure diagnosis and transplant journey.

In January 2019, Dennis was diagnosed with stage 3-colon cancer and is currently in remission. You can connect with Dennis at dtdt1123@gmail.com

Nicol McClendon

Nicol McClendon was born and raised in Hartford, CT. Nicol's love for writing came at a young age and continued throughout high school when she would pen short stories and poems that won awards and earned her many opportunities as a public speaker.

Following the murder of her first husband, Nicol found the strength to continue living through writing and traveling. Nicol became an author and entrepreneur when she published her first book; *It's My Story I Will Tell It - Pieces of Me.* She put a real face to hope and healing by sharing her uncensored truth about her journey through rejection, heartbreak and overcoming grief.

Nicol committed herself to helping others share their stories. She published a companion journal; *The Writers Journal – It's Your Story Tell It* to provide a guide for deepening the healing journey by allowing others to release their stories through expressive and reflective writing.

After her second husband was diagnosed with a terminal illness, Nicol co-authored the anthology; *Blessed Not Broken – Journey to Finding Purpose in Marriage, Motherhood & Entrepreneurship as a CEO Wife.*

Nicol is a bestselling author, emotional release writing coach, mother and a wife who will inspire you to open yourself up and pick up the shattered pieces of your life by continuing to believe in pure love and remembering the deep joy in living. You can connect with Nicol at authornicolmcclendon@gmail.com or visit her website www.nicolmcclendon.com

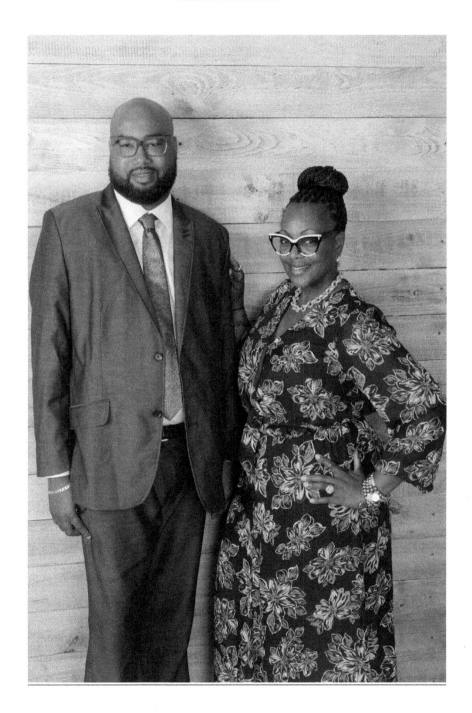

Dennis Thomas & Nicol McClendon

CPSIA information can be obtained
at www.ICGtesting.com
Printed in the USA
JSHW032240260922
31028JS00006B/73

9 781735 904603